# MIRA!

## David Soto Jr.

For Celia Martinez. I miss you and love you so much. I count the days until I dream of you next.

# Preface

The content in this book is not intended to be a substitute for professional medical advice, diagnosis, or treatment. Always seek the advice of your physician or other qualified health providers with any questions you may have regarding a medical condition. Never disregard professional medical advice or delay in seeking it because of something you have read in this book. Blah blah blah.

I get a lot of advice about making sure I have citations and stuff, that way people would take me seriously but that seems not at all like the kind of book I like to write. Most of the content in this book is either real life experience or my opinion. I did do some research and state some facts in this book but did it in such a general way that I don't feel citations were needed. That's the kind of writer I am. I break stuff down to the point that anyone can understand it and leave it up to the reader to research the subject further on their own if they want.

I feel I write for people who aren't prone to read medical studies, for people who want to just get to the good stuff without all the five-dollar words. I write this way because that's the kind of reader I am. People seem to like it. I was afraid that my first book, The Complete Guide to Primitive Eating, was too small and was lacking content but then the reviews started coming in. Turns out, the thing that I was afraid of was the very thing people praised the most.

I do have to tell you that this book pretty much exists because of Michael Pollan's *Omnivore's Dilemma*. This book was the source for a lot of my information on corn. It also sparked curiosity and lead to tons of research on other subjects, which I then added to Mira!.

I am not a professional by any means. I do not have a college education unless you count my Associates Degree in Mechanical and Electrical Technology from the Community College of the Air Force, which most people don't. I am not certified in anything. Nor do I have any letters in front of or after my name, unless Jr. counts. I am just an average guy who has read a lot of books, done a lot of research and conducted a lot of experiments on himself. My goal is to take all this information and put it in the hands of other average people out there like me, with hopes of helping them reach their goal.

I truly hope you enjoy this book.

David Soto Jr., Tucson, AZ

Introduction 8

Your Family Tree 14

Our Ancestors 18

The Problem Foods 23

What About the Kids 38

Chronic Inflammation & Disease 44

The Program 54

What are Latinas Saying? 65

What's Next? 74

About the Author 75

# Introduction

I used to get a lot of laughs when I did my George Lopez impressions. I did them so much that I can't even imitate my own grandmother anymore. I imitate George imitating his. "Allowance?! Mira, I allow you to live, cabrón!"

I was at a small birthday party a few years ago and, after a couple beers, I started letting the George Lopez impressions go. I had everybody rolling! People were laughing and having a good time. If the laughter would die down someone would mention something they remembered from one of his routines and then I would take over, doing the material with my best George Lopez accent. As the laughter continued I tried to think of the next joke I was going to tell and then I said this, "If your panza is bigger than your chi-chis, then it's time to do something." CRICKETS! It might as well have been a holocaust or 9/11 joke.

This happened way before I became the primitive guy but I never forgot it. The laughing stopped because every woman at that party could relate and they did not think it was funny. That let me know two things: Latinas having this big swollen stomach is common and they didn't like it, at all.

Not too long after that, I went to live in Mexico for a while. While I was there, the oldest daughter of the host mother I was staying with asked me about how to get rid of this. "This" was accompanied with a gesture of a back and forth movement of her hand on her stomach right below her rib cage with a combination frown and look of disgust. I was far from being the knowledgeable person I am today so, I really had nothing to say to her. But again, I didn't forget.

Then, four years later, I went back to Mexico for a month. I had learned a lot about nutrition by this time. Personally, I had been eating primitively for 3 years. I had a different mindset at the time and when I walked around the beautiful city of Guanajuato, Mexico I noticed swollen panzas everywhere.

This was not just something a few friends or relatives were suffering from, this was affecting most of the Latina population.

**What about the flacas?**

I didn't forget about you! Keep reading.

I remember someone telling me years ago, "Mexicans [Latinas} are fine as hell but you don't want to marry one. They eventually all get fat." Now this statement was made by a very ignorant young man and yes, it's very offensive but why would he say such a thing? The same reason why all stereotypes exist, because it is perceived as the truth. And, it perceived a truth because, in many of the cases, it is true. When people find out that I am 100% of Mexican origin they don't believe it. Why? Because I am 6'7". What is the stereotype about the stature of Mexican men? Well, I am proof that we are not all short but that doesn't mean a lot of us aren't.

So are all Latinas destined to get fat? Not necessarily, but I will say this — In my 40 plus years on this earth I have witnessed many Latinas, who were very thin as young ladies, lose their figure as they got older. But here is the thing, they didn't necessarily get fat. They got inflamed, swollen. Believe it or not, this has nothing to do with getting older.

Let me try to break it down to see if I can describe the situation. As a young lady, you had a thin or "nice" body. Some women may have even envied you. You ate whatever you wanted and always stayed thin. Then, in your late 20s and early 30s, you started to notice a change in your shape or even your weight. You start doing some crazy fad workout with your girlfriend and that seemed to help. You may have even gone on the occasional diet but essentially your eating habits never changed. In your late 30's and early 40, you are now two or three dress sizes bigger than you were when you were "young." You start to get frustrated because you can't stop the weight gain no matter how much you work out. You tried a diet here and there but those are only temporary and you fall back into your regular eating habits. In your 40's and 50's, you are now unrecognizable from your senior or wedding pictures. (With your big ass hair.) You may have diabetes or are taking some form of medication or two. Somewhere in between your 50s and 60s, your hospitalizations started. Does this describe you or anyone you know? Oh and if you had a baby in there somewhere, forget it!

So what happened? You just got older, right? Wrong. What is the one thing that stayed the same throughout the scenario described above? The food. You never stopped eating certain foods. Yeah, you gained some weight but what really affected the size of your clothes was chronic inflammation. Years and years of eating food that you are not designed to eat took its toll on your body. This caused your tissue, organs, and stomach to swell. This constant stress on your body had an effect on your metabolism and contributed to you storing fat. Did you get fat? Maybe, but not until years and years of chronic inflammation due to the foods you were eating.

## Mrs. Martinez.

My grandmother died in 2000 but I probably think about her every day. If not, then at least something I do every day is influenced by her, like my cooking style. Being her only grandson she spoiled me with food and gifts but mainly with love.

Being the oldest of 7 sisters, she was forced to quit school to help out around the house when her father abandoned his family. What does a woman do for a living without even having an elementary school education? As far as I can remember she made her living by cleaning houses. Even though she was the cleaning lady, everyone that she worked for loved her and had respect for her. They called her Mrs. Martinez.

She cleaned houses five days a week until breast cancer got a hold of her, then she dropped down to 2 or 3 days a week. She did that until she was absolutely too sick to clean anymore and stopped completely. Thus, her retirement years were spent sick and in and out of the hospital.

Family members traveled from afar to attend her funeral. Family, I didn't even know. Several of them got up to speak on her behalf. Through their sobs, they spoke of what an incredible woman she was and how she was so influential in their life. One very large, middle-aged man completely broke down when he relayed the story of how she bought him a bicycle for Christmas one year when he was a boy and how he could still hear her laughing as a result of seeing him ride that bicycle up and down the street.

With the knowledge that I have now, I could have helped her. If not prolong her life at least made those last years of her life more enjoyable. It's too late to help her but it's not too late to help you. If you are someone's mother or grandmother, my gift to your children or grandchildren is to keep you around a little bit longer, to improve the quality of your golden years. Yes, this book in honor of my grandmother but I have written it for you.

# Your Family Tree

I want you to look at your family tree. Look up and out to the sides. Look up and see your mom, your tias, and your abuelas. Look out to the sides at your sisters and your primas. My bet is most or all of them are one of two things: Overweight or Sick! Actually, if they are overweight, they are sick but I say one of the two for a very good reason. Being thin does not mean you are healthy. It may look more appealing to some but it doesn't mean that the person who is thin isn't struggling too.

Someone who is not overweight might be suffering from any of the following:

- Acne
- Eczema
- Irritable Bowel Syndrome
- Arthritis
- Crohn's Disease
- Chronic Sinus Infections

This list can go on. You may be wishing that you had their body but I am willing to bet they are wishing they didn't suffer from whatever ailment they have. I want you to try something. If there is someone in your family who is thin, someone who you wish you had their body and you think they are so lucky, ask them if anything is bothering them. Chances are they might be suffering from one of the ailments mentioned above. You just can't see it.

The reason I tell you to look at your family tree is because that is your future. These women share your very same DNA. The chances of you turning out like them are very likely. Is this what you want?

Though I am not a woman, if I look at the women in my family, this is what would I find:

- Obesity
- Diabetes
- High Blood Pressure
- Cancer
- Dementia
- Hospitalizations
- Medications
- Surgeries
- Some good ass cooking skills

So there is one thing on this list I want to have, the cooking skills. The rest, as my grandma would say, "Can go to hell!"

Because all these things are in my family tree I am very susceptible to suffering from them. Some of which, I already have. I have been obese and have had high blood pressure. And If I had continued on that path, I would be in the same boat as both of my grandmothers, slowly dying of diabetes.

But, just because I am prone to these things doesn't mean they have to happen. I can easily prevent any of them from happening to me by changing how I eat. THAT'S IT! And, I'm here to tell you that so can you. You have heard Einstein's definition of insanity, right? "Doing the same thing over and over again and expecting different results." This doesn't just apply to your shitty relationships. This can be applied to the world as a whole or to your family tree. Eat like your grandma and your mom and you will get the same results.

I say look up and out at your family tree because that is your future if you continue on your same path but now, I want you to look down. That's right, look at your daughters. What path are they on? Do they also fall in one of the two categories, sick or overweight? Do you want them to follow in the same footsteps as the rest of the women in your family?

I have recently learned the phrase "more is caught than taught." Rachel Cruise, daughter of financial guru Dave Ramsey, uses this phrase a lot in her book Smart Money Smart Kids. The premise is that you can't teach your children something you don't do yourself. Children learn by example. Have you ever thought, when I'm a mother I'm not going to (insert annoying thing you mother does here) and then one day find yourself doing or saying that EXACT thing? Not to long ago I found myself living in a house with my own little family for the first time in my life. And one day, having not heard the words in over 20 years, I said them; "Why are all these goddamn lights on and nobody is in here!" My god, I thought, I can't believe I just said that. My dad never taught me, "Son, this is how you bitch at your family about wasting electricity." He didn't need to. He set the example and, whether I wanted it to be or not, it was ingrained in my brain enough that I said those very words decades later when I came across my first opportunity to use them.

Whether you want to or not, you are leading by example. My question to you is, what kind of example are you setting?

# Our Ancestors

As Latinos, our ancestors were indigenous people, hunter-gatherers and we are of the same blood, the same DNA. Our bodies are not designed to eat many of the foods that are currently and readily available to us today. What happens when you give hunter-gatherers modern day processed food? Travel to a Native American reservation and take a look.

In 2006, I was activated to "protect the borders" and was sent to Arizona to man a post on the Tohono O'odham Nation. (Before you judge me for working on the U.S./Mexico border, a descendant of illegal immigrants myself, know that by volunteering, I took the place of someone who would be less compassionate. Like the one guy that actually brought his own rifle because he thought he would be hunting Mexicans.) Upon first arrival, someone asked how we were to tell the difference between the Tohono O'odham Nationals and Undocumented Immigrants. The answer was harsh and blunt but very true. "The Tohono O'odham Nationals will be the fat ones."

I am going to advise you to give up a lot of our traditional foods, like corn. I know what you are thinking. Latinos have corn in their blood! I have many responses to this.

— Latin America got into agriculture about 5000 years ago. Yes, this is a long time but compared to the time we humans have been on this earth, it's really not that long. Our species showed up here on earth about 200,000 years ago, our group, Homo, about 2 million years ago, and our original ancestors about 6 million years ago. To say farming is in our DNA might not be accurate.

— Let's just say agriculture is in our blood and that 5000 years of eating crops is enough time for our body to evolve to accept these domesticated plants as food. The problem is we aren't eating those crops that were produced 5000, 2500, 1000, or even 100 years ago. We are eating a modern day, mass produced, chemically engineered crops. Nothing like what our ancestors was growing. If corn is in our blood, it's not the corn you are eating today.

— My research shows that the staples in Latin American agriculture were squash, corn, beans, chiles, and potatoes. Nowhere could I find wheat or soy. The two crops that wreak the most havoc on our bodies today. (More on these later.)

— Even our ancestors knew corn was indigestible. That's why they processed it through nixtamalization. Nixtamalization is the process of cooking dried corn kernels over a long period of time in an alkaline solution of lime (the mineral, not the fruit) and ash. This process would dissolve the indigestible part of the corn and cause to swell up. A perfect example of this is the corn you find in pozole or menudo. Nixtamalization is still done but at an industrial level, far removed from the traditional methods are ancestors used and it is only done to the corn intended to make masa.

— How much corn, beans, squash, chili, and potatoes are you actually eating? This is mostly what our Aztec, Mayan, or Incan ancestors ate with the addition of some fish or meat. Is this what you mostly eat?

— Regardless of any of this I mentioned above, the thing that is KILLING us, the thing that our ancestors had very little access to, is sugar.

**The Sun**

If we want to mimic our ancestors we need to take a good look at the sun. No, not literally but think about it. The Mayans had Kinich Ahau, the Aztecs had Huitzilopochtli, and the Incas had Inti.

They all, to some extent, worshiped the sun and for good reason. The sun is the source of all life. Let me try to break it down.

The sun transfers it's energy to the grass through radiation hence the term, "rays" of sunshine. The grass takes that energy and uses it to grow tall. A cow comes along, eats that grass and converts its energy into protein. We then take the cow protein and make carne asada, converting the cow's energy into our own flesh and blood. This example is rudimentary at best. There are probably 1000s of other species of life forms that are actually affected in this one example. Not to mention the offsprings of both the cows and yourselves.

The sun provides life. Take if out of the equation and you have something completely unnatural, man-made. I bring the example of the cow because of an important factor. Most of the beef that you find at the grocery store came from cows that do not eat grass. They eat corn. Corn that is not made from energy from the sun but from fossil fuels. (More on this later.) The sun is taken out of the equation and therefore the beef you eat is no longer natural and that means neither are you.

Not only is the sun important to the food we eat it is important for us to come in contact with it. Our body turns the sun's rays into much-needed vitamin D. Can you imagine a life without sun exposure? Keep in mind that most of the pork and poultry you buy from the supermarket have lived such lives.

Everything our ancestors ate was a direct conversion of the sun's energy. Whether it was a vegetable or animal. Can you say the same about the food you eat now?

# The Problem Foods

## Wheat

Whether it is Whole or Raw, it is inedible. A kernel of wheat is made of three parts: The bran, the germ, and the endosperm. The endosperm, aka wheat gluten, is the pretty white part we make into bread. It is also the reproductive part of the plant. Like all living things, this plant wants to produce a surviving offspring. So, to protect its young, it covers the endosperm with the bran. The bran is indigestible so, even if the kernel is eaten, it can pass through the digestive tract intact. And, when it gets pooped out in the dirt, it's in a nearly perfect condition for it to sprout.

What we do as humans is separate the endosperm, the "edible" part, by processing it. We turn it into flour and then turn the flour into things like tortillas, sweet bread, and empanadas. What we are essentially doing is consuming something we would not be able to consume in nature and doing it in LARGE quantities.

I believe we all react negatively to wheat in some way. Some of us more than others. Just because you test negative for celiac, doesn't mean that test was accurate. I have read that the majority of the tests out there are inaccurate. Thus, people are being sent home from the doctor's office after being told they are not allergic, so they can, and do, continue to eat wheat. They also stay sick.

Your body doesn't see wheat as food (because it's not). It sees it as bacteria, so your white blood cells attack it. This causes inflammation, and a swelling in your gut that Dr. William Davis calls a "Wheat Belly." I have seen one of my client's waistlines shrink inches in just 30 days, having only lost five pounds. Why the drastic loss of inches but not a drastic loss in weight? He gave up wheat and the swelling simply went down.

Wheat is addictive. I know someone who was sick. All of her symptoms were signs classic gluten intolerance. She had been sick for years and has seen several doctors during this time. She was frustrated and tired of feeling ill. I advised her to go gluten-free. She tried it but found it to be difficult. She found that if she just ate a little, bit she actually felt better. That folks, is called withdrawal. Gliadin, a protein found in wheat and other grains, has been said to have an opiate effect on the brain. When you give it up abruptly you will experience withdrawal. In my opinion, if your body throws a fit because it has to go without something it's used to, that is an addiction. Generally speaking, if something is addictive, it's not good for you. Am I right? Cigarettes, crack, sugar, heroin, booze? I can not find any health benefit of consuming gluten. Maybe I haven't done enough research. If you happen to come across something, please send it my way.

Wheat raises your blood sugar higher than sugar! Have you heard of the Glycemic Index? The Glycemic Index is used to measure how much specific foods increase you blood sugar levels, otherwise known as blood glucose. Depending on which chart you look at, white bread will be higher than whole wheat or vice versa, but on most charts you will see that both are actually higher than table sugar! Yet the government recommends a diet in whole grains.

## Legumes

This one has been very controversial lately. People love their beans, especially Latinos. In fact, beans are considered an important part of Latin American agriculture as it is one of the "Tres Hermanas" along with corn and squash.

Granted there are some nutritional benefits to eating beans but let's look and some of the drawbacks.

Lectins. Lectins are one of the things that can damage the lining of the small intestine. That being said, One of the main reasons for omitting all of the foods I am suggesting you eliminate is to allow your gut to heal.

Phytic acid. This prevents any nutrients that legumes may have from actually being absorbed by the body.

FODMAPs. FODMAP stands for Fermentable Oligosaccharides, Disaccharides, Monosaccharides And Polyols, which are a cause of major IBS symptoms such as gas, pain, and diarrhea. Remember the old playground tune: "Beans, Beans, They're good for you heart. The more you eat the more you fart?"

It's important to know that the two most damaging "foods" that fall under the category of legumes are peanuts and soy. (More on soy below.)

Just like all the other foods on this list. You can reintroduce them later and see how they make you feel. I tried to reintroduce beans once because I read in a book that it was good for helping you lose weight. It only took a couple meals for me to realize my body did not react well to beans. I still avoid them to this day. You may react differently but first, let's get that gut healed up.

**Soy**

Soy is the number-one genetically modified organism in the U.S. It is basically created in a lab and mass produced in the fields. This is not food. Not even close. When you eat soy you are eating something that cannot be found in nature. If you know me as @primitivedave, you know that this is enough reason for me not to eat soy but let's look a little further into it.

First, keep in mind that soy is a bean, aka a legume, and I just got done telling you that legumes can damage the lining of the small intestine. This can lead to intestinal permeability and chronic inflammation. (More on chronic inflammation later.)

Next, soy contains a high concentration of phytoestrogens. Phytoestrogens act as estrogen in the body. The overconsumption of soy can lead to what is know as Estrogen Dominance or Estrogen Toxicity.

I am certainly no expert in the area of estrogen but a little research on the internet yielded this long list of estrogen toxicity symptoms.

- Breast tenderness
- Depression, fatigue, poor concentration
- Endometriosis
- Fibrocystic Breast
- PMS

- Fibroids
- Water retention and bloating
- Fat gain around hips and thighs
- Breast and Uterine Cancer
- Difficulty losing weight
- Infertility
- Irregular menstrual periods
- Low sex drive, low libido

Any of these seem familiar?

## Dairy

I like to base everything I talk about on what comes most natural to us as humans. Does drinking milk from another animal's breast seem natural? Think about it. Why would one species drink the milk created by another species? Whale milk is made for whales. Dog milk is made for dogs. Human milk is made for humans. And cow milk is made for cows.

Dairy is an irritant that leads to chronic inflammation and autoimmune disorders (I cover later in this book). Personally, too much dairy leads to excess mucus production, upset stomach, and acne. Let's look at the two ingredients in milk that contribute to these symptoms: lactose and casein.

### Lactose

Most of us can't digest lactose. We stop producing the enzyme that helps digest it soon after infancy. It makes sense, doesn't it? This would be about the time we would have been weaned off of our mother's breast.

Words that end in "-ose" indicate that they are a sugar. Eg. Fructose, glucose, and sucrose. The word lactose simply means, milk sugar. I cover the negative effects of sugar below and in the section of this book covering diabetes.

**Casein**

Casein has been linked to autism and type one diabetes. These two diseases are formed in infancy. Do you understand this? The very thing you are giving your children could be the cause of two life-long conditions.

Casein has an opiate effect thanks to casomorphins. Guess where there is a high concentration of casein? CHEESE! Does the word casein sound familiar? Say it with me, queso. This is why my heart starts racing at the thought of a quesadilla!

Milk is pasteurized and homogenized. Most of the nutrients in it are destroyed in these processes. The chemical structure of the milk is changed when it is pasteurized and homogenized. It's basically not even milk anymore. This is a big factor as to why dairy is such a gut irritant.

### Sugar

I cover the negative effects of sugar extensively in the diabetes section of this book so, what I want to do here is take a common sense look at how unnatural it is for us to eat sugar.

How much sugar do you think our ancestors had access too?

Every living creature has one goal and that is to produce a surviving offspring. This includes plants. Some plants protect the seed of their offspring by covering it with and indigestible coating, such as wheat. Others protect it with biotoxins, such as potatoes and tomatoes. Some use the flavor of bitterness as a warning not to eat them. In the case of fruit like berries, it's the opposite. They want to be eaten so they can be passed through the digestive system a dropped at another location to sprout and grow. This is why berries are bright in color and sweet.

When it comes to foraging for food out in the wild, if something is bitter, it is a good indication not to eat it. However if something is sweet, your body instinctively gives the green light to eat it. You see, sugar is not easily found in nature. Your body knows this so, when you introduce something sweet into your body it goes nuts. Your body says, eat as much of this while you can.

This point was really made clear to me when I watched Out of the Wild — Venezuela. In this show, 9 strangers were dropped in the middle of nowhere Venezuela and had to walk out, over 70 miles, with limited supplies and no food. After just a couple days, they were starving. But unlike other survival shows, they didn't just have to survive for a few days and wait to be rescued, they had to walk out. A few quit but the rest pressed on, killing a foraging whatever they could to eat. The scene I remember the most like I was there myself, was the one where they were walking one day and stumbled across a patch of wild blueberries. Like animals, they dropped to their knees and went wild picking and eating the berries.

I can't think of a better example of our human survival instincts kicking in. Their body told them to "eat as much as you can." Why? 1) They were mobile. They needed the energy to continue to walk. Also, because they were walking to safety, this meant they had to eventually leave. They had to fill up and go. The same would go if you came across a clean source of water in this situation. 2) The berries were a rare find. They had gone days without seeing any. Who knows when they would see another patch. 3) The berries were sweet. This let them know they were safe to eat. This isn't a theory on how our ancestors reacted to sugar. This is a real life accounting of how humans reacted to sugar in 2010.

Now, imagine this instinctive reaction to sugar when you are at a restaurant, your home, or the grocery store! Sugar is not so hard to find now. The grocery store is full of isle upon isle of it. Your cupboards are full of it too. It is so available that you don't even have to chew to get it. You can just pour it into your body in the form of juices, soda, and caramel lattes. How are are you supposed to turn off this instinct to "eat as much as you can?" In the wild, you didn't have to. You would either leave where the sugar was available or you would simply run out. But, in this day and age, these two scenarios are nearly impossible.

A perfect, real world scenario: Have you ever been to a Native American reservation? If you have, you may have noticed a syringe disposal container in every public bathroom. This is an indicator of how common diabetes is among indigenous people. This is what happens when you introduce sugar into a community of hunter-gatherers.

**Grains**

This is another controversial topic. The reason for this is that we have been told for 60 years that we should be consuming a large quantity of grains and food made from grains.

In 1956, the U.S. Government started recommending the Four Basic Food Groups. They were fruits and vegetables, dairy, meat, and grains. Depending on your age, you may remember this being taught to us in elementary school. In 1992, the U.S. implemented the Food Pyramid. At the base of the Food Pyramid, the largest portion was the recommendation of 6-11 servings of grains, cereal, bread, and pasta. Though there was a slight change to the Food Pyramid in 2005, it held strong until 2011 when it was replaced with My Plate. My Plate is essentially a pie chart depicting that 30% of your plate should contain grains. For 60 years the U.S. Government has been programming us to eat grains. No wonder so many people have issues with being told not to eat them. Guess which branch of the government is responsible for putting out the all of this information over the past 6 decades? The U.S. Department of AGRICULTURE!

I see two major issues with the USDA's recommendations.

1) Some grains like white rice and wheat flour can raise your blood sugar more that a serving of actual table sugar will. A constant high blood sugar can lead to several health problems. Ones I am sure you are familiar with. I go into detail on this in the diabetes section of this book.

2) Grains like wheat, rye, and barley contain gluten. The consumption of gluten can lead to inflammation and a long list of associated diseases. I cover these diseases in great detail in an upcoming chapter.

Do you know what ranchers feed cattle to make them fat? GRAINS! They feed them grains for this specific reason. It makes them fat and it will do the same to you! This realization alone was enough for me to give up grains. No science needed here. Not for me anyway!

**Corn**

First off, remember how I said soy was the number one genetically modified organism? Well, corn is number two! (FYI, cotton is number three but we don't eat cotton so, I guess it's cool.)

As a people, corn is an important part of our history. For centuries, our ancestors lived off corn. It was a staple food for us. "Food" being the key word here. You see, corn is no longer a "food" it is a "commodity," a raw material that can be bought and sold.

When Che Guevara tried to buy corn from the local farmers of Bolivia during his attempt to lead a revolution, to feed his guerrilla army, he was met with resistance. Why? Corn was a food, not a commodity. Farmers could not feed their families with money. Their "choclo" was not for sale and thus, not a commodity.

Corn is no longer food, therefore, the tortillas so commonly consumed among the Latinos of North America are also no longer food. There are two major events in history that contribute to this, the end of World War II and The North American Free Trade Agreement.

Corn is a very nitrogen needy crop. Back in the day, U.S. farmers would not grow corn more than two seasons in a row on the same plot of land within a 5 year period because corn would rob the soil the much-needed nitrogen, not to mention the insects and disease it would bring. Farmers would have to rotate the crops with soybeans. The natural process of growing soybeans utilizing the sun would make the soil, once again, nitrogen rich.

Enter the end of WWII. A surplus of Ammonium Nitrate that was manufactured for munitions was repurposed as fertilizer. This fertilizer supplied the corn with its much-needed nitrogen and farmers could now grow corn season after season. And because corn was more profitable, due to government subsidies, they did.

What you have to realize here is the nitrogen supplied by Ammonium Nitrate is synthetic, man-made. The natural process the involves the sun was replaced with a chemical process the used natural gas instead, essentially making corn petroleum based. Take this and the fact that corn has been genetically modified over the years to produce a higher yield, resist pesticides, or even produce their own pesticide, makes corn completely unnatural.

Corn cost more to grow than it does to sell. So why do U.S. farmers grow so much corn? Because the government makes up the difference by paying the farmers subsidies. This means that whoever buys the corn from the farmer is getting it super cheap. This leads to a stockpile of corn. What do you do with tons and tons of corn sitting around? Well you can make it into a sweetener (High Fructose Corn Syrup), cooking oil, fuel for your car, or you can sell it to Mexico. When the North American Free Trade Agreement (NAFTA) was implemented on January 1, 1994, this is exactly what happened. Not only did the completely synthetic corn find it's way into Mexico, but because it was so cheap, it lowered the value of corn grown in Mexico.

# What About the Kids

I hear a lot of excuses from women when I talk to them about cleaning up their diets and eating healthy. The most common ones have to do with their kids.

Excuse 1: I don't have time to prepare a meal for me and then another for my kids.

Excuse 2: I don't want to deprive my kids of anything just because I have to eat this way.

Ok Mama, are you ready for this? You are the one in charge! You are making the food. They eat what you make or they don't eat. It's that simple.

Zig Ziglar used to tell a story about a man that had a beautiful dog. When Zig saw this dog he was blown away by how thick and shiny the dog's coat was. Zig ask the owner, "What do you feed him?" "Turnip greens," responded the owner. "Turnip greens? I didn't know dogs would eat turnip greens." "This one wouldn't," said the owner, "not for the first two weeks."

When your kids have no other option, they will eventually eat what you make. You are not neglecting your kids by not feeding them dinosaur shaped chicken nuggets. In fact, you are doing quite the opposite. You are doing your jobs, as mothers, by making the right choices for them. You don't let your kids play in the street or stay out all night regardless of how much they want to. Why? Because you know what's good for them. Now, with a little bit of help from me, you'll know what's good for them nutritionally.

You are not depriving them of anything. They need nutritious food to grow and develop. It's not like I'm telling you to make some crazy gross tasting fad diet food. You can serve them Arroz con Pollo but without tortillas or the use corn oil. Or, make them hamburgers with lettuce instead of buns.

### Which came first?

I know how easy it is to appease your children when they are throwing a fit because they want a cookie. If you give them that cookie they will shut the hell up for a while but what if that cookie is the actual cause of the problem? You ever wonder why kids act like little crackheads when it comes to sugary snacks and why they are so happy when they get what they want?

There are experts out there that say that ADHD is directly linked to the amount of sugar and wheat your children eat. Dr. David Perlmutter and Dr. Joseph Mercola are just two of them. Also, a quick search of the internet will lead you to thousands of articles and studies linking the connection. Many of them via the National Center for Biotechnology Information, one of the most commonly referred to websites for people who want the straight up facts about a medical topic.

You can spend hours researching this subject but, why bother. What does your gut tell you? What does common sense tell you? What does your experience tell you? Personally, I have seen a parent feed their child waffles topped with peanut butter and maple syrup and then immediately follow it up with their daily prescription drug to counteract the effects that were to come. Do you think that if there is a connection to a child's behavior and a pill there would also be a connection to their behavior anything else they put in their mouth?

**The New Diabetes.**

Growing up with a sick grandmother my mother, the nurse, made sure I knew of her medical conditions so that I could report it to emergency personnel if the situation were ever to arise. One of the things I knew to report was that she was a diabetic. "What kind of diabetes does she have?" my mother asked me. "Uhh, I don't know", I responded. "She has Adult Onset Diabetes."

Have you heard of Adult Onset Diabetes? If you haven't, there is a good reason for that. It's now commonly called Type II Diabetes. This is simply due to the fact that it so common in children that they can no longer call it Adult Onset Diabetes.

Do you understand this? What used to take decades to damage the pancreas now only takes years and as a result, more and more children are getting it. You, as a mother and grandmother, have the ability to change this and that's by simply saying, "no."

**What about outside if the home?**

A common concern heard is, well I don't want my child to get sick if they are exposed to it outside of the house so, I give them some at home. Robb Wolf once addressed this in an episode of his podcast. I think I recall him saying, "That is effing stupid!" He followed up with something to the effect of, "Well, might get exposed to cocaine. Should you give them some of that too?" I know this is a little extreme but you get the point.

In fact, since you know they are going to get exposed to foods like wheat and sugar, why not minimize the effects of the exposure by providing them with super healthy immune systems by not feeding them crappy foods in your home. Also, by teaching them that junk food is not good for them in your home, where they eat most of their meals, you will be empowering them to make better decisions on their own when not at home. Just like you would with drugs and alcohol or even having good manners.

Remember you have no control over what your child does outside of your home. You can only teach them, by example, to make good decisions when you are not around.

**Foods that make you grow.**

I had the privilege of being a part-time father figure to a little girl for a short time. She was well behaved and rarely sick. This had a lot to do with what we fed her at home but she also made good decisions when she wasn't around us. How did we do it? We ate healthy meals together every day but most of all we didn't demonize the bad foods we didn't want her to eat. This was done by breaking food down into two groups: foods that helped her grow and foods that didn't. It was as simple as that.

You'd be amazed at what a child will and will not eat once they have learned what will help them grow and what will not. We would get reports back from her grandparents and other relatives on the foods she passed up on because they would not help her grow.

Now, she did like sweets but it seemed only because it was the thing to do like what I witnessed at a birthday party once. It was cupcake time and she was not about to be the only one not to get a cupcake. We let her have it and after two bites she was done and back to playing with her friends. We didn't tell her she couldn't have it. We didn't have to.

# Chronic Inflammation & Disease

Inflammation is your body's way of healing itself. There are two types: Acute and Chronic

## Acute Inflammation

You have more than likely experienced acute inflammation when you sprained your ankle or got stung by a bee. The result is the affected area can become swollen, red, painful, or even warm. Typically these effects go away over a short period of time when the threat is gone. If the inflammation persists, it is a good indication that something more serious is actually wrong. People who thought their wrist was sprained often find out it is actually broken after the swelling does not go away after a couple days.

## Chronic Inflammation

Chronic inflammation affects your body in the same way as acute inflammation (pain, swelling, redness, and heat) but is present over a long duration of time, months or even YEARS. Imagine your body's reaction to a bee sting never going away. Now imagine this bee sting happening inside your body where it is kind of hidden. (It's not hidden for a lot of you but more on this later.)

Now, what causes chronic inflammation? There is a lot of science out there that answers this question and I'm not going go lie, some of it is way over my head. Let me try and break it down for you.

**1)** Chronic inflammation can be a result of an autoimmune response or disorder. This is when your immune system attacks healthy tissue, mistaking it for infectious agents. Examples of this are Crohn's disease, celiac disease, and irritable bowel syndrome. Now, what causes this response? Intestinal permeability. Intestinal permeability is basically holes in the protective lining of your intestinal tract. These holes allow, well, shit to leak out of your gut and into the rest of your body. Hint: Shit is not supposed to be anywhere but your intestine!

What causes these holes in your gut? The most common answer I have found in my research is Gliadin, which is found in wheat. (memmer?) Other foods that have evidence of causing leaky gut are (can you guess?) grains, legumes (like peanuts and soy), and sugar. Stress and medications are also well-known contributors.

**Note:** If you consider your immune system an army, and you have an autoimmune disorder, your soldiers are constantly in a war. A war that doesn't exist. If all your soldiers are busy fighting a pretend war, what happens when there is a real invader? You get sick. Ever wonder why some people are never sick and some people seem to always get sick? We are all exposed to the same germs. It's just that for some of us, our army is standing by ready to engage in battle while for others, they already are.

**2)** The other cause for chronic inflammation is a steady, low-intensity irritant. This is the real killer. It's doing people harm and they don't even know it. So for those people who are like, I don't have Crohn's disease or I was tested for Celiac and I don't have it, they are worse off. Because they are not diagnosed with a disease they feel they are free to eat cake or whatever and, as a result, they maintain a low level of inflammation over years or even decades.

Below is a list of the top ten causes of death in the United States in order:

1) Heart disease
2) Cancer

3) Chronic lower respiratory disease
4) Stroke
5) Accidents
6) Alzheimer's disease
7) Diabetes
8) Influenza and pneumonia
9) Kidney disease
10) Suicide

Guess how many of these, according to the Centers for Disease Control and Prevention in 2011, are attributed chronic inflammation? Seven! Heart disease, cancer, chronic lower respiratory disease, stroke, Alzheimer's disease, diabetes, and kidney disease are all a result can all be directly linked chronic inflammation.

What can be considered a low-intensity irritant? All of the foods I am trying to get you to stop eating in the book, which happens to be the same foods linked to intestinal permeability mentioned above. Other irritants can be alcohol, medications like non-steroidal anti-inflammatory drugs (aspirin, ibuprofen, and naproxen), tobacco, and stress.

**Note:** Non-steroidal anti-inflammatory drugs (NSAIDs) have been linked to gastrointestinal damage (Hmmm), heart disease and stroke (Number one and number four from the above list). The evidence is so blatant that the Food and Drug Administration has pulled numerous prescription NSAIDs off the market and requires warning labels on the over the counter ones, with the exception of aspirin.

**Food Baby**

People who eat the way I eat tend to hang out together, especially online. A very common thing I have seen over the years is people posting pictures of the inflamed gut, most commonly called a food baby or gluten baby. These posts come from people who don't eat wheat but sometimes, whether intentional or not, get "glutened." This "baby" is irritation caused by gluten, which is the source of the Gliadin I mentioned earlier. For most of the people, including me, the swelling and irritation goes away after a couple days or so.

Now this reaction would be considered acute inflammation, but what if one were to wheat again at their next meal or the next day and the next and the next? This would result in chronic inflammation. What is your diet like? Are you eating, what can be considered, a minor irritant? How often?

**Got that "itis?"**

Chronic inflammation can also be attributed to any disease or condition that ends in "itis." Below are some of the most common ones:

• Rheumatoid arthritis

- Osteoarthritis
- Periodontitis
- Hashimoto's thyroiditis
- Sinusitis
- Ulcerative colitis

Guess what's commonly prescribed to people who suffer from arthritis? NSAIDs! If you haven't caught on here, arthritis is a result of chronic inflammation. NSAIDs cause chronic inflammation! Therefore, the taking of NSAIDs are actually making the condition worse, not better.

## The Bee Sting

Remember the bee sting I mentioned earlier? If you or anyone you know has ever been stung by a bee, then you may have seen how much swelling it caused. This is inflammation in action. Now, imagine your internal organs having the same reaction because of the irritants you consume.

I want you to keep in mind that your heart and lungs are protected by your ribcage. They are also separated from the rest of your internal organs by a wall of muscle known as the diaphragm. Your diaphragm basically lies horizontally right at the bottom of your rib cage. Right below your diaphragm is your liver and stomach. Now if these two organs swell up, where do you think they are going to go? Not up. You diaphragm prevents that. How about down? Nope, your other organs take up the rest of the space in your thoracic cavity. The only option is OUT! This is your panza.

You may or may not have excess body fat but if you have a belly, especially right below your rib cage, I am willing to bet a big part of that is inflamed organs.

You can exercise and restrict your calories all you want but if you are still eating irritating foods, neither will reduce the inflammation in your gut. This is why so many of you go on diets or start strenuous workout routines, only to get disappointing results. Any results that you do see are either minor or temporary.

## Diabetes

Diabetes is so common now that, according to a nurse friend of mine, when people are asked, "How is your blood sugar?" people are responding, "Oh not bad. It's around 200." Hello! This is not "not bad" this is double of what's normal. DOUBLE! Also, this same nurse tells me that when she asks patients if they have any conditions that she needs to know about they often respond with "no" even though they have diabetes. This is a disease! It is so common, though, that people seem to accept it. Let me tell you, it's not ok! Diabetes will guarantee you one of two things, an early death or a miserable last 10 to 20 years of your life.

When you eat a donut, the sugar and the flour cause your blood sugar levels to spike, almost immediately. This signals your pancreas to release insulin so it can do its job, which is to regulate your blood sugar levels by delivering the sugar to your muscles and liver in the form or glycogen. (If these glycogen stores are full, the insulin carries the sugar to fat cells for storage making the fat cells larger and you fatter.) If you eat another donut or wash it down with a latte, this process continues. Taxing your pancreas like this may not be so bad on occasion but if it happens every day, meal after meal, you are going to develop problems.

Problem 1: Your liver and muscles no longer respond to the insulin. They become resistant and tell insulin to bugger off. This is known as "Insulin Resistance" and can be an indicator of, or lead to, prediabetes.

Problem 2: Your pancreas says, screw it. After years of trying to regulate your blood sugar, your pancreas will eventually just call it quits. When this happens, congratulations, you're diabetic.

Problem 3: High blood sugar, which can affect anything that relies on blood flow in order to work. These are some of the best parts of your body. These include your eyes, your kidneys, your heart, your feet and your brain.

Diabetes is number 7 on this list of top ten causes of death in the United States mentioned above. The funny thing is, it leads to four other causes of death on that very same list. Number 1: Heart Disease, Number 4: Stroke, Number 6: Alzheimer's, and Number 9: Kidney Disease. Type II diabetes is not something that should be taken as lightly as it is. The messed up part about it, it's completely preventable.

# The Program

## Introduction

What you are about to read is a modified version of my program, The Complete Guide to Primitive Eating. The Complete Guide to Primitive Eating is dedicated to slowly eliminating all the problem foods mentioned in this book as well as developing some habits you may need to make this a complete lifestyle change. If you think this is something you may need, I suggest you follow the link I provided and download it right away. In the least, check out the reviews.

This program is designed to eliminate certain foods over a long period of time, at your own pace. This is a no-pressure method. If you get stuck at a step, keep working on it until you've mastered it. There is no timeline, so you won't fall behind. This is not a challenge so there is no chance of failing. Take your time.

Once you get past this introduction, simply read the first step. Once you have met the requirements for mastering it, read the next step and move on when you are ready. When you move on to step two, you will continue with what you have just eliminated in step one, and so on and so forth. You will continue this process until you reach the last step. Once at this point, you will have developed several life-changing habits, one at a time, at your own pace.

Are you ready?

### Step 1: No Mas Tortillas, At Least The Flour Ones... for now!

Basically, kiss your quesadillas and burritos goodbye. What's that, you don't eat quesadillas or burritos? Well, it's time to give up sandwiches, too! In fact, toast, rolls, and bagels are out too. That's right, you are giving up bread. I KNOW! I have heard it all before, so I don't need to hear how much you love bread. I don't care.

How do I do it? It's called a lettuce wrap. Many restaurants, like Five Guys and Jimmy Johns, will wrap meat and cheese in lettuce at no extra cost. All you have to do is ask. If a place won't do it, just ask for it sans bun and eat it with a dang fork! Or better yet, order a steak!

This step is important because chances are, you consume most of your wheat via tortillas or bread. Later we are going to eliminate wheat so, consider this a baby step. Doing this will take a lot of stress off of going gluten-free.

If you are trying to lose weight, eliminating bread will make a significant difference in your body fat. This step alone will be a giant leap towards regulating your blood sugar levels and controlling your insulin spikes. Imagine eating a juicy rib-eye with grilled veggies at your local steak house, but passing on the rolls. You will not only omit your normal rapid spike in insulin, (which causes your body to store fat) you will also avoid that bloated-and-then-tired feeling afterward. Chances are, you probably eat the equivalent of calories in bread to your meal before your entree even comes. You will walk away from meals feeling just as satisfied but without having consumed all those extra, no purpose, calories.

You have mastered this step when it is a part of your daily practice and you're feeling good about it. Keep in mind, this could take a couple weeks

## Step 2: Stop Eating Breakfast

No, I am not about to make you skip breakfast but you are about to skip the conventional breakfast food. In this step, you will be learning that breakfast doesn't have to consist of your typical breakfast foods. Cereal, hash browns, omelets, and waffles are out. Anything else is in. So get out last night's leftovers and heat them up because you are not having breakfast for breakfast for a while.

Chances are your current breakfast habits are killing you. Consuming  sugar and food that turn into sugar, first thing in the morning is detrimental to your health. These "meals" will raise your blood sugar, drain your energy, and make you hungry just a few hours later. Is this really how you want to start your day?

This step is important because the next step is a biggie and doing this one is going to make it that much easier.

You have mastered this step when you have done this it for 7 consecutive days in a row. You can resume eating breakfast foods but you are going to find that as you move on to the next step you are going to be very limited in what you can eat. I have two words for you: Bacon and Eggs.

### Step 3: Go Gluten Free

Going gluten-free is not easy but the rewards are incredible. From now on, consider yourself gluten-free. This means no wheat, rye, or barley products. Bread, tortillas, cereals, pancakes, and waffles are already out of your diet. Those were all stepping stones to this step. Now, you have to cut out the pasta and sweets made with flour.

You are going to have to start looking for gluten in your food that isn't an obvious wheat product. Here's a good example. I thought soy sauce, of all things, would be gluten free. I mean, it's SOY sauce for Pete's sake. One day I took a look at the label and, lo and behold, there it was, plain as day: WHEAT. If you're looking for a gluten-free soy sauce, try Tamari or even better Coconut Aminos. Soy will be off the menu in a couple weeks anyway.

In the future, you will not be eating anything labeled "gluten-free." Anything labeled as such is usually processed junk, BUT if it is going to make your transition a little easier, I will allow some gluten-free products. Just keep in mind, if you are trying to drop some excess pounds of fat, that the wheat flour substitutes commonly found in gluten-free products will cause you to store fat nearly as much as wheat flour will. Brown rice flour may not have all the side effects as wheat flour, but it has one: It makes you fat and that's a pretty important side effect. Be wary of anything labeled "Gluten-free!" Eat a steak instead.

Cross contamination is something to look out for. Take this example: You find out your favorite chicken wing joint has a food allergy menu online. You check it out and find that most of their flavored wings are actually gluten-free. Great, right? Let's go down to have a cider and some hot wings. The problem is this place fries their wings in the same oil they fry their onion rings, breaded chicken strips, and boneless wings in (which are also breaded). Sad news friend, your wings are not gluten-free.

This could be, by far, the hardest step you are going to have to get through but the benefits are going to be the greatest. This could take you the longest to get a hold of. Don't be surprised if this takes a month.

You have mastered this habit when it seems like second nature and you are past any withdrawal stages.

### Step 4: Go Soy and Peanut Free

This may not seem like that big of a deal but keep in mind that products made from these items are also on the list. This will include peanut butter, soy sauce, chocolate, and certain vegetable oils.

You are going to have to really pay attention to food labels here. I have often had to spend several minutes looking for a ready made marinara sauce that wasn't made with soybean oil. They do exist. The good ones are made with olive oil instead.

You have mastered this habit when you have gone soy and peanut free for 14 consecutive days.

### Step 5: Go Dairy Free

Here is another toughie. Up until now you have probably been enjoying milk, ice cream, and, more likely than anything else, CHEESE. It's time to let it go. From this point forward, you are now Dairy Free.

You have mastered this habit when you have gone dairy free for 14 consecutive days. You will probably feel a lot better and even look a bit slimmer.

### Step 6: Go Sugar Free

This one is going to hurt, but it's time to go sugar free. And yeah, I mean all sugars and even artificial sweeteners. Table sugar, honey, maple syrup, agave nectar, stevia, equal, and basically any ingredient that ends in "ose." Those "gluten-free" treats, like cookies, they go bye-bye. Take note, that I am not saying "carbs." I am saying SUGAR.

Also, I know you're not going to like this but, fruit is included in this step. Once your blood sugar is under control and you have reached your goal weight, fruit can be added back to your grocery list. Whole fruit only, though. Smoothies are not allowed back in.

You have mastered this habit when you have gone sugar free for 21 consecutive days

### Step 9: Go Corn Free

Yep, it's time to give up the traditional staple of our people. From now on no more corn tortillas, elote, choclo, and anything else that has corn in it. Again it's very important that you pay attention to food labels. Corn is in everything! It's usually in the form of High Fructose Corn Syrup (HFCS), which you should have already eliminated, but keep an eye out for corn starch and corn meal. There is actually a long list of other ingredients that are made from corn but you eliminated most of them when you went sugar free.

Remember, we are trying to heal your body specifically, your gut. Eliminated corn is a very important part of this.

You have mastered this habit when you have gone corn free for 14 consecutive days

### Step 8: Go Grain and Legume free. (Optional)

This step, right here, is the major difference between the program I am setting up for you

(Latinas) and <u>The Complete Guide to Primitive Eating</u>.

In The Complete Guide to Primitive Eating, there is no Soy and Peanut Free step only a Legume Free step, which, soy and peanut are both a part of. Legumes are anything that comes in a pod. This includes pinto beans, lentils, black beans, and garbanzo beans. Since beans are a major part of Latinos diet, and the damage they cause varies on the individual and how they are prepared, I have made it optional. Soy and peanuts are very damaging, though, so I gave them their own step.

In The Complete Guide to Primitive Eating, there is no Corn Free step. Since corn is a grain, it is included in the Grain Free step but, again, rice is a staple food, and since white rice is known to be very tolerable, I have made this alteration to the program.

This step is your call but I want you to be very smart about it. Since you have started this program you have eliminated the most common causes of chronic inflammation and diabetes and have, no doubt, seen some major improvements in your health but if you are still suffering from symptoms like bloating, other digestion problems, skin issues, or still have some pounds to lose, you may want to take this step on.

You have mastered this habit when you have gone grain and legume free for 14 consecutive days.

Now that you have made it this far, how do you feel?

In the end, this is all that matters but yeah, I know, some of you want to look good too? Well, how do you look? Another thing to pay attention is how are you performing? Are you no longer sleepy at work? Are you no longer exhausted after a long day on the job? Do you have more energy to tend to your children or grandchildren?

Seriously, I want to know. You can send me a message at dave@theprimitiveyou.com.

**Try it, if you want but…**

When this is all said and done and you are feeling healthy and looking good, you may want to try to reintroduce some of these foods back in. I say go for it but I want you to LISTEN TO YOUR BODY. Your body will, almost immediately, tell you that you are not ready to reintroduce something. You may experience gas, bloating, diarrhea, pain, an overall feeling of blah. This is where you are going to have to experiment. I can't say what you will tolerate and what you won't. Everyone is different.

On a trip to Mexico one year, my girlfriend at the time and I thought we would reintroduce corn into our diet in the form of tacos and quesadillas. I did pretty well on it but she was having some serious negative reactions to it. In the end, we found out that she would do better with flour tortillas than she did with corn. After the trip, we both went back to our regular gluten and corn free diet.

# What are Latinas Saying?

The way I see it, I have two things working against me:

1) Is there any proof that any of the things I talk about in this book actually work?
2) I wrote a book on women's health and I am a man.

I knew this when I started writing this book, so I reached out to the Latinas that I knew, and even ones that I didn't. I was hoping that someone would contribute to this book by telling their story, thus solving the two problems I mentioned above. I waited for months and no one responded. Then I created a little survey and posted it on www.mirathebook.com. Slowly but surely, they started coming in. Below you will see all the responses that I have received so far. As they come in, I will continue to update electronic version this book. When I get enough input, I'll publish it in paperback.

This is the most important part of the book. The real life evidence from Latinas that their health and life changed for the better when they made some changes in their diet.

If you want to be in this very book you are reading, please visit www.mirathebook.com to find a link to the survey. I look forward to hearing how your life has changed.

# Marah
**Colorado Springs, CO, USA**

**Which foods have you reduced drastically or eliminated from your diet, even if temporarily, for at least 21 days or more at a time?**

- Pastries
- Added Sugar
- Soda
- Milk
- Cheese
- Dairy
- Peanuts

**Which food listed above had the most DRASTIC effect on your body when you eliminated it?**

Animal products (Dairy, Milk, & Cheese), and bad fats mostly

**Where did you notice improvements after eliminating the foods you did?**

- Energy Levels
- Weight
- Dress Size
- Skin
- Sleep
- Digestion
- Sugar Cravings
- Mood

**Tell me a little more about one or more of these improvements. Which one was the most drastic, the one you never thought you would see, or had the biggest impact on your life?**

The biggest impact I have seen is in my children. I have a 19-year-old who was raised eating like "a Mexican"... we used to eat all sorts of bad stuff. I changed my diet and lifestyle in 2006, and my daughter was born a year later. She is now 8 years old and she is healthy and fit and my son was a bit overweight for most of his childhood. I now see the difference it has made, my daughter doesn't know what McDonalds taste like, she doesn't eat junk often. In fact, she will crave the greens and nuts as snacks. Although my son was 11 when I started this change, it still has taken him some time to change his habits. I hope I have shown my kids that the change can have positive effects on your body and overall health.

**If you had a chance to say something to all the sick and obese Latinas out there, who were looking for help, what would you say to them about making the changes you made to your diet.**

I say this very often - change is hard because you see it as such. Change can be educational, delicious, inexpensive, exciting, motivational and can produce ripples with the rest of your family. It has to start somewhere and you are that someone!

You can learn more about Marah at www.marahsshop.com.

# Veronica
**Tucson, AZ, USA**

**Which foods have you reduced drastically or eliminated from your diet, even if temporarily, for at least 21 days or more at a time?**

- Bread

- Corn Tortillas
- Flour Tortillas
- Pastries
- Rice
- Legumes (Beans)
- Wheat
- Grains
- Added Sugar
- Soda
- Cereal
- Milk
- Corn
- Soy
- Peanuts

**Which food listed above had the most DRASTIC effect on your body when you eliminated it?**

Wheat, flour, corn, added sugar, pastries, corn, grains

**Where did you notice improvements after eliminating the foods you did?**

- Energy Levels
- Weight
- Dress Size
- Skin
- Sleep
- Digestion

- Sugar Cravings
- Mood

**Tell me a little more about one or more of these improvements. Which one was the most drastic, the one you never thought you would see, or had the biggest impact on your life?**

David and I had been friends for a number of years. When I saw his body and lifestyle start to transform for the better, I had to ask him what he was doing. As a person who has tried every fad diet out there, I noticed David had lost weight, was able to keep it off, and was toning up! He began spending much more time outdoors and started to demonstrate a healthier lifestyle that I was interested in. Since following David and beginning to eat Primitively, the biggest impact I have noticed is my digestion. As soon as I eliminated wheat, flour, and grains (which were the first to go), I noted a big improvement in my digestion. I was digesting food regularly, having daily bowel movements, and oddly enough, no more gas, bloating or constipation (great news for a woman). I have also noted that when I try to cheat and eat these things, my digestion is impacted within hours. Instantly, I feel constipated and bloated. I have taken this as it is a clear sign from my body asking me not to consume these products anymore. I like and feel relieved that Primitive eating asks you to know what you are putting into your body:

preservatives, harmful chemicals, pesticides, antibiotics...the list goes on! I am a label reader now!! I am terrified of what the FDA deems 'safe,' and the dangerous effects these products will have on our later lives. I can see the direct cause and effect of certain foods when I have eliminated them and then tried to consume them again: dairy (bloating, digestion problems, and nasal drip), sugar (same symptoms). I used to have problems with acne, now my face has cleared up. In fact, I get so many compliments on the appearance of my skin it's surprising! Others call it "radiant, perfect, and clear!" People now ask me what I am doing to lose weight and stay healthy. I consider Primitive Eating much more a lifestyle than a diet. I can eat when I want, still enjoy foods (sometimes I modify recipes!), and have incorporated much more movement into my lifestyle. The results are that I feel better, look better, have lost weight, kept it off, and feel relieved knowing what I am consuming in my diet. I look forward to eating this way for the rest of my life, and remaining healthy until my old age! David has always been responsive and helpful in guidance and answers to my questions. Thanks David for your hard work, passion, and inspiration!

**If you had a chance to say something to all the sick and obese Latinas out there, who were looking for help, what would you say to them about making the changes you made to your diet.**

David's video "No Mas Tortillas" really hit home for me. Just on my mother's side (I'm full Mexican by the way), my abuela passed from cancer, my mom is overweight and has type 2 Diabetes, and four out of her five siblings have serious health-related issues (overweight, kidney issues, diabetes, and various major surgeries). What's your math, how many of your family members are sick and overweight? The insight that this video helped me see was that, 1) I am going to end up just like them unless I do something different, and 2) the common denominators of all of these illnesses has to be food and lack of movement. As soon as I started to live Primitively, I lost weight and my health improved. This meant no more tortillas, menudo, pan dulce, frijoles, quesadillas. If you read and follow David's research you will see that these foods are actually making you and all of our Latina friends and family SICK! No, this doesn't mean that I don't eat these foods, or can't still enjoy them, I just modify their recipes if I can. Meatless tacos with all the filings, posole, and menudo without the hominy, I can still have tamarindo, piña, mango and jicama with lime and chili! But, no mas tortillas or pan dulce. They are killing yo, literally, slowly, and miserably. I had a man tell me not too long ago that when he was younger, a friend of his gave him a piece of advice about Latina women. "Be warned that when you marry a Latina, look at her mother, that's exactly how she'll end up looking." Ouch!! Now, go look at your tias, your mama, your nana, is that what you want to end up looking and feeling like? Not me, and I won't if I continue to eat Primitively. David, and I, and many others, are proof that Latinos can still be Latinos without having to live and eat in a way that is harmful to them. This is a lifestyle that is important to your longevity, peace, and usefulness. It is the only 'diet' that has EVER worked for me!

# What's Next?

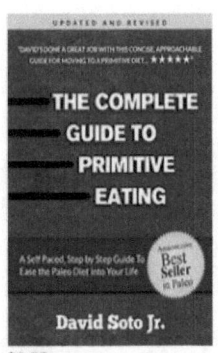
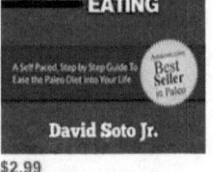

$2.99
Kindle Edition

$2.99
Kindle Edition

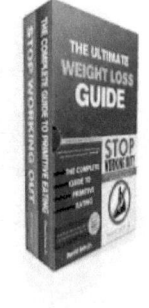

$3.99
Kindle Edition

If you like what you just read, please check out my other books on Amazon and please leave a review for this one while you are there. It will really help spread the word. If you didn't like it, never mind. ;-)

This will be the last of my health and wellness books for a while. I am moving on to writing my memoirs, *The Second Time I Lost My Virginity and Other Love Stories,* as well as some fiction. If you like my work and am interested in any upcoming books I may release, please join my readers list at www.davidsotojr.info

# About the Author

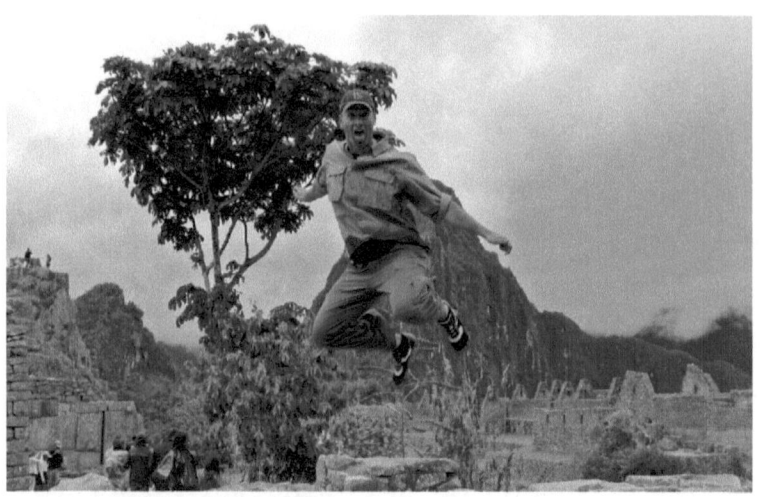

David was born in Gardena, California and spent most of his childhood in Los Angeles. In high school, his family moved to a small town in Missouri. At age 17, David joined the Air Force and spent the next 23 years toggling between active duty Air Force and the Missouri Air National Guard. In 2002 he was deployed under Operation Enduring Freedom and in 2004 he served his country, as a civilian contractor, in Iraq.

Throughout the years, when not in uniform, David tried his best to fit into society. He got a job, went into debt to buy a house and a car, and tried to find a girl to marry and start a family with. None of these seemed to work out for him. Instead, he felt best on the road. At the age of 30, he sold most of his possessions, put his house up for rent, hit the road, and (more or less) hasn't stopped since.

David writes, speaks, and coaches clients on how to regain their freedom through simplification. He calls it: Getting Primitive. You can learn more about his philosophy at www.theprimitiveyou.com.

www.ingramcontent.com/pod-product-compliance
Lightning Source LLC
Chambersburg PA
CBHW050512290526
45786CB00007B/2534